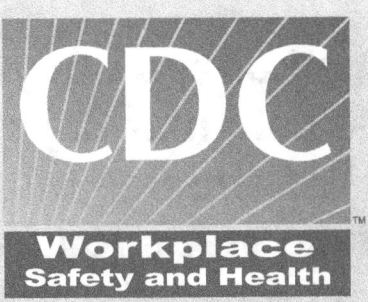

Workplace Safety and Health

Evaluation of Cancer and Magnetic Fields in an Office

Kenneth W. Fent, PhD
Elena Page, MD, MPH

Health Hazard Evaluation Report
HETA 2008-0286-3084
County of Guilford, Information Services
Department
Greensboro, North Carolina
May 2009

DEPARTMENT OF HEALTH AND HUMAN SERVICES
Centers for Disease Control and Prevention

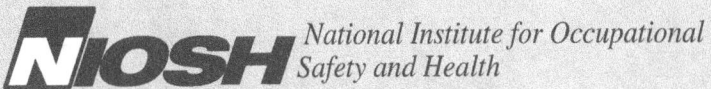

National Institute for Occupational
Safety and Health

The employer shall post a copy of this report for a period of 30 calendar days at or near the workplace(s) of affected employees. The employer shall take steps to insure that the posted determinations are not altered, defaced, or covered by other material during such period. [37 FR 23640, November 7, 1972, as amended at 45 FR 2653, January 14, 1980].

CONTENTS

ABBREVIATIONS

ACGIH®	American Conference of Governmental Industrial Hygienists
amp	Ampere
CU	Chilling unit
EMF	Electromagnetic field
ft²	Square feet
GM	Geometric mean
GSD	Geometric standard deviation
Hz	Hertz
IARC	International Agency for Research on Cancer
MF	Magnetic field
mG	Milligauss
NIOSH	National Institute for Occupational Safety and Health
NIEHS	National Institute of Environmental Health Sciences
OEL	Occupational exposure limit
OSHA	Occupational Safety and Health Administration
pCi/L	PicoCuries per liter of air
PDU	Power distributing unit
PEL	Permissible exposure limit
REL	Recommended exposure limit
SD	Standard deviation
STEL	Short term exposure limit
TLV®	Threshold Limit Value
TWA	Time-weighted average
WEEL	Workplace environmental exposure limit
WHO	World Health Organization

What NIOSH Did

- We looked at cancer diagnoses surveys from current and former Information Services Department employees. The Public Health Department provided these surveys.

- We measured MFs around electrical devices in the facility.

- We measured eight employees' personal exposures to MFs.

- We presented our findings about the cancer diagnoses to employees.

What NIOSH Found

- The numbers and types of cancer reported did not appear unusual. The reported cancers were unlikely related to MFs or other workplace exposures.

- The highest MF levels were found in the computer server room, ranging from 0.5 to 1000 milligauss (mG). The main MF sources were electrical panels, power distributing units, and chilling units.

- Average personal MF exposure levels ranged from 0.43 to 2.7 mG. These levels were well below related occupational exposure limits. Two employees who worked in the computer server room, printing room, operations room, and envelope stuffing room had the highest personal MF exposures of 1.3 and 2.7 mG.

- Two peak personal exposures from the computer server room were at or above the American Conference of Governmental Industrial Hygienists ceiling limit of 1000 mG. This limit is for employees with cardiac pacemakers or similar medical devices.

What Managers Can Do

- Encourage employees to learn about cancer risk factors, steps to reduce risk for preventable cancers, and cancer screening programs.

- Restrict employees with electronic medical devices, such as cardiac pacemakers, from entering the computer server room. This room contains sources of MFs that could exceed the recommended limit for such people.

- To further reduce MF exposures, limit the amount of time employees spend in the computer server room and encourage employees to increase their distance from MF sources.

What Employees Can Do

- Learn about cancer risk factors, steps to reduce risk for preventable cancers, and cancer screening programs.

- Learn about MF exposures and report any MF concerns to management.

The National Institute for Occupational Safety and Health (NIOSH) received a request for technical assistance from the County of Guilford, Public Health Department in North Carolina. The request concerned cancer among employees in the Information Services Department. Employees were concerned about exposure to magnetic fields (MFs) from computer servers and other electrical equipment at the worksite. A survey of workplace MFs was conducted in November 2008.

SUMMARY

The numbers and types of cancer reported among Information Services Department employees did not appear unusual. Reported cancers were unlikely related to workplace exposures. The highest MF levels were found in the computer server room near the electrical panel, PDUs, and CUs. Personal MF exposures were well below applicable OELs, but can be reduced further by limiting the amount of time spent near the primary sources of MFs. Employees with cardiac pacemakers or other electronic medical devices should not access the computer server room due to the potential for interfering MFs.

On November 12–13, 2008, we conducted a survey at the County of Guilford, Information Services Department in response to a technical assistance request submitted by the County of Guilford, Public Health Department in Greensboro, North Carolina. The request concerned a possible cancer excess among Information Services Department employees. Employees were concerned about MF exposures in the workplace and the potential association with cancer. We reviewed cancer diagnoses surveys from current and former Information Services Department employees that the County of Guilford, Public Health Department provided. We also measured the MFs throughout the workplace, particularly in and around the computer server room. Personal MF monitoring was conducted on eight employees who worked in different locations in the workplace. Two of the employees worked in the computer server room and adjacent areas (printing room, operations room, and envelope stuffing room).

The numbers and types of cancer reported among employees did not appear unusual, and the cancers were unlikely related to workplace exposures. The MF levels ranged from 0.5 to 1000 mG in the computer server room, with the highest levels occurring near the electrical panel, PDUs, and CUs. The two employees working in the computer server room and adjacent areas had GM personal exposures of 1.3 and 2.7 mG. All other office employees had GM personal exposures below 1.0 mG. Except for a Computer Operator with a GM exposure of 2.7 mG, all monitored employees had GM exposures below those for employees in similar job categories. Two peak personal exposures were at or above the ACGIH ceiling limit of 1000 mG for employees with cardiac pacemakers or similar electronic medical devices. Both of these peak exposures were traced back to computer server room activities.

Employees with cardiac pacemakers or other electronic medical devices should not access the computer server room because of the potential for MF interference with the function of their medical devices. For all other employees, personal MF exposures measured in this survey were well below applicable OELs. Nevertheless, MF exposures can be reduced by limiting the amount of time spent in the computer server room and by increasing working distance from MF sources.

Keywords: NAICS 921110 (Executive Offices) EMF, magnetic fields, executive offices, computer programming, computer server, cancer

On September 16, 2008, NIOSH received a request for technical assistance from the County of Guilford, Public Health Department in Greensboro, North Carolina. The request concerned a possible excess of cancer among employees at the County of Guilford, Information Services Department. The employees were concerned about MF exposures emanating from the computer servers and other electrical equipment in the workplace and their potential association with cancer.

On November 12–13, 2008, we made a site visit to the County of Guilford, Information Services Department. We met with management and employee representatives and observed work processes, practices, and workplace conditions. Our findings regarding the occurrence of cancer among Information Services Department employees were presented at an open meeting for all employees. We measured MFs in the computer server room and other workplace areas and asked eight employees to wear personal monitoring devices to measure their MF exposures throughout the day. A closing conference was held with management and employee representatives to summarize site visit activities and provide preliminary findings.

Workplace Description

The County of Guilford, Information Services Department is at 201 North Eugene Street in Greensboro, North Carolina. The building was originally constructed as a department store in 1948. The County of Guilford acquired the building for government use in 1989, and the Information Services Department moved into the building in 1991. The Information Services Department occupies approximately 23,000 ft² of the basement. The computer servers are housed in a 3,240 ft² room. The printing room, operations room, and envelope stuffing room are adjacent to the computer server room (Figure 1). These rooms contain electrical equipment such as printers, computer controls, tape drives, and an envelope stuffing machine. The Information Services Department employees provide information technology and computing services to the County of Guilford. Currently 52 employees work in the Information Services Department; since 1990, 151 employees have worked there.

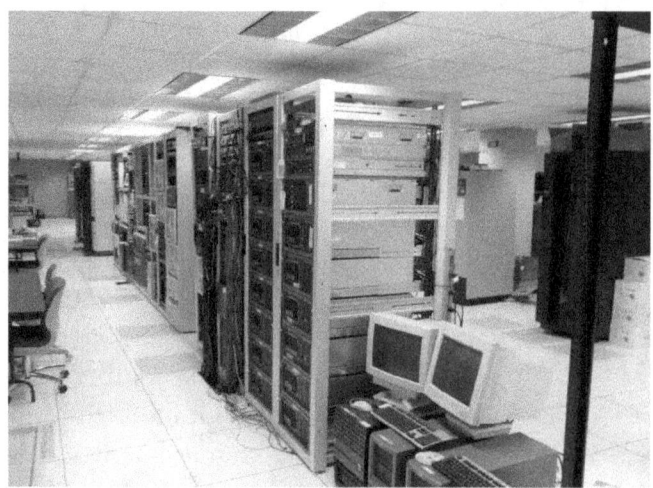

Figure 1. Computer server room

ASSESSMENT

Prior to our visit, the Public Health Department had conducted a survey to determine the number of Information Services Department employees who had been diagnosed with cancer. This survey was sent to all current employees and to those employees who had left the department in the past 5 years (an additional 30 employees). A summary of these surveys was sent to NIOSH. Along with reviewing this summary, we called two current employees who were reported to have been diagnosed with cancer but who did not submit a survey.

The Public Health Department had conducted various tests in response to employee concerns and provided us with the results. We reviewed the results of an indoor environmental quality survey conducted on June 26–27, 2008, by the Workplace Group, a consultant hired by the county. We examined reports of water quality testing performed by the North Carolina Laboratory of Public Health on September 10, 2008, and results of five radon tests performed by the Radon Testing Corporation of America in July and August 2008. We also reviewed the material safety data sheet for the insecticide used by the pest control contractor in the building.

We monitored MFs from 5 to 2000 Hz, a frequency range that encompasses the electrical power frequency of 60 Hz. For this evaluation, MFs were measured in mG. Another common unit of measurement is microTesla (1 microTesla equals 10 mG). The

ASSESSMENT

(CONTINUED)

methods used to collect area and personal MF measurements are described in Appendix A. In addition, monitored employees were asked to complete a job-task log sheet on which they recorded any tasks involving trips to the computer server room or the use of electrical equipment other than typical office equipment. The employees in the computer server room were not asked to complete the job-task log sheet due to the complex nature of their work. Appendix B discusses the OELs and potential health effects from MF exposures.

RESULTS

Cancer

Current employees returned 39 surveys, former employees returned 10, and the Public Health Department reported one deceased person with cancer. Seven employees reported being diagnosed with cancer since 2002, three with breast cancer, one with pancreatic cancer, one with lung cancer, one with nonmelanoma skin cancer, and one with cancer of the appendix. The mean age of those diagnosed with cancer was 55, and the mean age of those without cancer was 48. The employees diagnosed with lung and pancreatic cancer had been cigarette smokers.

MF Area Measurements

More than 80 area MF measurements were collected throughout the work area with particular emphasis in the computer server room and adjacent areas, which included the printing room, operations room, and envelope stuffing room. Table 1 provides a summary of the area measurements. Appendix C, Figure 2 shows the location and magnitude of the area measurements collected in the computer server room and adjacent areas.

Health Hazard Evaluation Report 2008-0286-3084   *Page 3*

Table 1. Magnetic field area measurements

Room / area	Range of measurements (mG)	Sources of MFs greater than 10 mG
Computer server room	0.5 – 1000	Electrical panel, PDUs, CUs
Printing room	3.0 – 20	Printer, CU
Operations room	0.5 – 12	Tape drive
Envelope stuffing room	0.5 – 8	None
Backup battery room	40 – 700	Electrical panels, PDUs, CUs
Office areas	0.3 – 200	Paper shredders, portable heaters

Measurements in the computer server room ranged from 0.5 to 1000 mG. The highest level in the computer server room was measured within an inch of the electrical panel containing a 1000 amp circuit breaker. In the computer server room MF measurements up to 30 mG near the CUs and 300 mG near the PDUs were measured. Measurements above 10 mG were also recorded at a printer in the printing room and a tape drive in the operations room. The MF levels in the backup battery room, an area in which employees did not typically spend much time, ranged between 40 and 700 mG. The highest levels (150 to 700 mG) in the backup battery room were measured near the electrical panels. Measurements in the office areas were generally 0.6 mG or less and are similar to levels measured in other office environments [WHO 2007]. Higher levels were observed near electrical equipment. For example, 200 mG was recorded near an operating paper shredder in office 024. However, this MF level fell to 0.4 mG when the paper shredder was turned off. A portable heater in office 016 emitted 40 mG during operation but only 0.5 mG when turned off.

MF Personal Measurements

Eight employees wore personal monitors during the morning hours. Appendix C, Figure 3 shows the work station locations of the monitored employees. Appendix C, Figures 4 through 11 show personal MF exposures over time, as well as summary statistics for those personal exposures. A summary of the personal MF exposures is presented in Table 2. Because the data are positively skewed (greater number of low MF levels compared to relatively high MF levels), the GM and GSD are the best measures of central tendency and scatter. The two employees who worked in the computer server room and adjacent areas (printing room, operations room, and envelope stuffing room) had the highest GMs and GSDs. Aside from one instance in which the Programmer walked under an outdoor power transformer (Appendix C, Figure 4), all exposures over 100 mG were traced back to job tasks in the computer server room or adjacent areas using the job-task log sheets. These exposures are indicated in Appendix C, Figures 4 through 11.

Table 2. Magnetic field personal monitoring results

Job title	Work station	Sampling time (min)	MF levels (mG)			
			Minimum	Maximum	GM	GSD
Chief Information Officer	Office 017	194	0.14	1000	0.56	1.8
Information Security Specialist	Office 037	178	0.11	35	0.60	1.8
Programmer	Office 041	215	0.01	550	0.44	2.0
Senior Software Architect	Office 043	182	0.11	250	0.81	3.0
Computer Operator	Server area	188	0.11	5600	2.70	6.1
Operations Manager	Server area	244	0.14	420	1.30	3.1
Web Applications Manager	Office 047	243	0.14	28	1.00	1.8
Administrator	Office 050D	175	0.14	180	0.55	2.6

In this section, we discuss our findings on cancer and MFs at the County of Guilford, Information Services Department. Information is provided on breast, lung, and pancreatic cancer; cancer clusters; and MF exposures measured in this evaluation. The most frequently diagnosed cancer type among the current and former employees of the Information Services Department was breast cancer, which is the most common cancer in women in the United States, affecting one of eight women [American Cancer Society 2008a]. Lung cancer is the second most common type of cancer among men and women in the United States. Other types of cancer diagnosed were pancreatic and nonmelanoma skin cancer, which are also common, and cancer of the appendix, which is less common.

Breast Cancer

An estimated 178,480 cases of invasive breast cancer were diagnosed in women in the United States in 2008, making it the most common cancer in women in the United States [American Cancer Society 2008a]. Although epidemiologic studies have identified some factors that appear to be related to increased risk for breast cancer, much remains unknown about its causes. Well-established risk factors include family history of breast cancer, biopsy-confirmed atypical hyperplasia, early menarche, late menopause, postmenopausal hormone replacement therapy, not having children or having the first child after 30, alcohol consumption, overweight or obesity (especially after menopause), never breastfeeding a child, low physical activity levels, and higher levels of education and socioeconomic status [American Cancer Society 2008a]. Breast cancer is not known to be associated with environmental or occupational exposures other than high doses of ionizing radiation [Goldberg and Labrèche 1996; Weiderpass et al. 1999; Carmichael et al. 2003]. The risk is highest if exposure occurs during childhood and is negligible after age 40. Several studies have found teachers and other professional and managerial employees to have an increased risk for developing breast cancer [Rubin et al. 1993; King et al. 1994; Pollán and Gustavsson 1999; Bernstein et al. 2002; Snedeker 2006; MacArthur et al. 2007]; but others have not [Coogan et al. 1996; Calle et al. 1998; Petralia et al. 1998]. No causative workplace exposures have been identified for these occupations, and it is postulated that the possible increase in risk is a result of nonoccupational risk factors such as parity (number of times a woman has given birth), maternal age at first birth, contraceptive use, diet, and physical activity [Threlfall et al. 1985; Snedeker 2006; MacArthur et al. 2007]. Women with higher educational status are also more likely to have mammograms, thus increasing detection of breast cancer. A recent study compared the incidence of invasive breast cancer among women who were screened once between ages 50 and 64 to women screened three times between ages 50 and 64. Distribution of known risk factors was similar between the two groups, but the rate of invasive breast cancer was 22% lower in the group screened only once, suggesting that some breast cancers regress without treatment [Zahl et al. 2008].

Lung Cancer

Lung cancer is the most common cause of cancer death in both men and women. An estimated 215,020 new cases of lung cancer were diagnosed in 2008 [American Cancer Society 2008b]. The most significant risk factor for lung cancer is cigarette smoking, which accounts for 87% of cases in men and 85% in women [Miller 2000]. Radon is the most common cause of lung cancer in nonsmokers, and second most common cause of lung cancer overall, accounting for more than 20,000 cases of lung cancer annually in the United States. Almost 3,000 of these 20,000 cases occur in people who have never smoked [EPA 2008]. Secondhand smoke is the third most common cause of lung cancer in the United States, with more than 3,000 cases annually [American Cancer Society 2008c; EPA 2008]. Known occupational causes of lung cancer include asbestos, arsenic, chromium, nickel, cadmium, coke oven emissions, tars, and soot [American Cancer Society 2006].

Pancreatic Cancer

The lifetime risk of having pancreatic cancer is about 1 in 76. An estimated 37,680 new cases of pancreatic cancer were diagnosed in 2008, and about 34,290 died of the disease. The most significant risk factor for pancreatic cancer is cigarette smoking; 20 to 30% of cases are likely due to smoking. Chewing tobacco also increases risk. Other risk factors include being African-American, obesity, sedentary lifestyle, diabetes, chronic pancreatitis, and cirrhosis of the liver. Pancreatic cancer has no proven occupational causes, but heavy exposure to pesticides and dyes is a suspected cause [American Cancer Society 2008d].

Cancer Clusters

Because of the concerns among the Information Services Department employees about cancer, it is helpful to review some general information about cancer and the approach we take in determining whether cancers have any relationship to the workplace. Cancer is a group of different diseases that have the same feature, the uncontrolled growth and spread of abnormal cells. Each different type of cancer may have its own set of causes. Cancer is common in the United States. One of every four deaths in the United States is from cancer. Among adults, cancer is more frequent among men than women, and it is more frequent with increasing age.

Many factors play a role in the development of cancer. The importance of these factors varies for different types of cancer. Most cancers are caused by a combination of several factors. Some of the factors include (1) personal characteristics such as age, sex, and race; (2) family history of cancer; (3) diet; (4) personal habits such as cigarette smoking and alcohol consumption; (5) the presence of certain medical conditions; (6) exposure to cancer-causing agents in the environment; and (7) exposure to cancer-causing agents in the workplace. In many cases, these factors may act together or in sequence to cause cancer. Although some causes of some types of cancer are known, we do not know everything about the causes of cancer.

Cancers often appear to occur in clusters, which scientists define as an unusual concentration of cancer cases in a defined area or time [CDC 1990]. A cluster also occurs when the cancers are found among employees of a different age group or sex than is usual. The cases of cancer may have a common cause or may be the coincidental occurrence of unrelated causes. The number of cases may seem high, particularly among the small group of people who have something in common with the cases, such as working in the same building. Although the occurrence of a disease may be random, diseases often are not distributed randomly in the population, and clusters of disease may arise by chance alone [Metz and McGuinness 1997]. In many workplaces the number of cases is small. This makes detecting whether the cases have a common cause difficult, especially when no apparent cancer-causing exposures are present. It is common for the borders of the "cluster" to be drawn around where the cases of cancer are, instead of defining the population and geographic area first. This often leads to "clusters" that are not real.

DISCUSSION
(CONTINUED)

When cancer in a workplace is described, learning whether the type of cancer is a primary cancer or a metastasis (spread of the primary cancer into other organs) is important. Only primary cancers are used to investigate a cancer cluster. To assess whether the cancers among employees could be related to occupational exposures, we consider the number of cancer cases, the types of cancer, the likelihood of exposures to potential cancer-causing agents, and the timing of the diagnosis of cancer in relation to the exposure. These issues are discussed below in a series of questions that relate to this request.

Do Information Services Department employees have more cancer than people who do not work in the Information Services Department?

Even though comparing the cancer rate among Information Services Department employees to a standard population is difficult, the number of cancer cases among current and former employees does not appear to be excessive. Because cancer is a common disease, it may be found among people at any workplace. In the United States, one in two men and one in three women will develop cancer during their lifetimes. This does not include basal or squamous cell skin cancers, which are very common (more than 1 million diagnosed annually), or any in-situ carcinomas other than bladder. If these were included, rates would be even higher. When several cases of cancer occur in a workplace they may be part of a true cluster when the number is greater than we expect compared to other groups of people similar in age, sex, and race. Disease or tumor rates, however, are highly variable in small populations and rarely match the overall rate for a larger area, such as the state, so that for any given time period some populations have rates above the overall rate and others have rates below the overall rate. So, even when a higher rate occurs, this may be completely consistent with the expected random variability. In addition, calculations like this make many assumptions that may not be appropriate for every workplace. Comparing rates without adjusting for age, sex, or other population characteristics assumes that such characteristics are the same in the workplace as in the larger population, which may not be true. However, general information on cancer rates is useful for providing perspective on the cancers in your population.

Do the Information Services Department employees have an unusual distribution of types of cancer?

No. Five different types of cancer were diagnosed among employees of the Information Services Department. Cancer clusters thought to be related to a workplace exposure usually consist of the same types of cancer. When several cases of the same type of cancer occur and that type is not common in the general population, it is more likely that an occupational exposure is involved. When the cluster consists of multiple types of cancer without one type predominating, then an occupational cause of the cluster is less likely.

Is exposure to a specific chemical or physical agent known or suspected of causing cancer occurring in the Information Services Department?

This is unlikely. The relationship between some agents and certain cancers has been well established. For other agents and cancers, there is a suspicion, but the evidence is not definitive. When a known or suspected cancer-causing agent is present and the types of cancer occurring have been linked with these exposures in other settings, we are more likely to make the connection between cancer and a workplace exposure. Radon is known to cause lung cancer, but radon levels were very low, ranging from 0.1 to 0.5 pCi/L. The Environmental Protection Agency recommends taking action if levels are above 4 pCi/L. The average indoor radon level is about 1.3 pCi/L, and the average outdoor level is about 0.4 pCi/L. Office buildings usually do not have significant hazardous exposures, and we did not identify any chemical or physical agents based on our review of the previous indoor environmental quality report, water testing, or from our walk-through surveys of the Information Services Department that would link potential work place exposures to the reported cancers.

The association between EMFs and various cancers has been the subject of intense research for many years. In 2002, IARC classified extremely low frequency MFs as possibly carcinogenic to humans, based mainly on studies of residential exposure to extremely low frequency MFs and childhood leukemia [IARC 2002]. An update of this evaluation published in 2007 did not change the classification based upon more recent studies [WHO 2007]. This report states that the evidence for an association between female breast cancer and extremely low frequency MFs was considerably weakened, does not support an association, and that the evidence is sufficient to "give confidence that MFs do not cause" breast cancer. In addition, the report states that the association between breast cancer and extremely low frequency MFs should be given low priority for further research. Other recent studies have reached similar conclusions [Feychting and Forssen 2006; Kheifets et al. 2008].

Has enough time passed since exposure began?

If we suspect that cancers may be related to workplace exposures based upon an apparent excess of cancer or an unusual distribution of cancer, and we identify agents we suspect of causing the cancer, then we look at latency periods. Latency periods are the time between first exposure to a cancer-causing agent and clinical recognition of the disease. Latency periods vary by cancer type but usually are a minimum of 10 to 12 years [Rugo 2004]. For example, it can take up to 30 years after exposure to asbestos for mesothelioma to develop. Because of this, past exposures are more relevant than current exposures as potential causes of cancers occurring in employees today. Because there was no apparent excess of cancer, an unusual distribution of cancer, or any hazardous exposures noted among Information Services Department employees, the issue of latency is not relevant.

Electric and Magnetic Fields

The term radiation is commonly used to refer to ionizing radiation, which is energy that is able to ionize atoms or molecules of the substance in which the energy is absorbed. This causes chemical changes that damage tissues and structural materials in the body. Nonionizing radiation refers to the lower energy forms of the EMF spectrum such as radio waves, microwaves, infrared, and visible light, and does not carry enough energy to ionize atoms or molecules.

EMF radiation is composed of both electric fields and MFs. Electric fields are produced by voltage and increase in strength as the voltage increases. MFs result from the flow of current through wires or electrical devices and increase in strength as the current increases. Electric fields were not monitored during this survey

DISCUSSION
(CONTINUED)

because they are shielded or weakened by materials that conduct electricity, even materials that conduct poorly, including building materials and human skin [NIEHS 2002]. In contrast, MFs are not easily shielded and can pass through the human body, where they could potentially affect biological systems.

Personal exposures measured in this survey did not exceed the ACGIH TLV ceiling of 10000 mG. This and other recommended OELs for MF exposures are based on acute effects, such as induced currents in cells or nerve stimulation, which are known to occur at high exposures—more than 1,000 times higher than MF levels typically found in occupational settings [NIEHS 2002]. More information on OELs and health effects related to MF exposures is provided in Appendix B.

Extremely low frequency MFs are ubiquitous because they are present wherever there is electricity. However, the amount of extremely low frequency MFs in the environment has increased due to electricity demand, advancing technology, and changes in work practices [WHO 2002]. Extremely low frequency MFs range from 3 to 3000 Hz with most exposure coming from the power-line frequency of 50 to 60 Hz. Exposure to MFs in homes is relatively consistent throughout the world, with GMs between 0.55 and 1.1 mG [WHO 2007]. Occupational exposure can be much higher, with exposures up to 100 mG near electrical conductors. MF exposures average 4 to 6 mG for electricians and electrical engineers, 10 mG for power-line employees, and above 30 mG for welders, railway engine drivers, and sewing machine operators [WHO 2007].

MF levels decrease with increasing distance from the source. Although 40 mG was measured at a portable heater in room 016 during operation, 0.4 mG was measured at the desk just a few feet away. A level of 150 mG a few inches from a PDU in the computer server room decreased to 30 mG at a distance of 2 feet, and dropped to 8 mG at 8 feet.

According to the job exposure matrix for power-line frequency MFs [Bowman et al. 2008], the GM exposures for computer operators and programmers are 1.7 mG and 1.0 mG, respectively. Exposures to the Computer Operator and Operations Manager in this survey may be compared to the GM for computer operators, while exposures to the other employees may be compared to the GM for computer programmers (Table 2). With the exception of

DISCUSSION
(CONTINUED)

the Computer Operator, exposures in this survey are below the GM levels measured for similar job categories in other workplace studies [Bowman et al. 2008] and therefore may be considered typical for this type of work environment.

The Computer Operator performed a variety of job functions in the computer server room and adjacent areas, including printing, envelope stuffing, and server maintenance. Many of the Computer Operator's exposures (Appendix C, Figure 11) were greater than 25 mG, including several of prolonged duration (>10 minutes). The Computer Operator had a spike in MF exposure of 5600 mG (Appendix C, Figure 11). According to the area measurements, this exposure most likely occurred in the computer server room, and may have occurred near the electrical panel. This peak exposure was above the ACGIH recommended ceiling limit of 1000 mG for employees with cardiac pacemakers or other similar electronic medical devices [ACGIH 2008]. In addition, the peak exposure for the Chief Information Officer (Appendix C, Figure 6), which was traced back to the computer server room, was at the ACGIH ceiling limit of 1000 mG [ACGIH 2008]. This ceiling limit is intended to prevent MF interference with electronic medical devices.

CONCLUSIONS

We found no evidence that the cancers reported are associated with work in the Information Services Department because the number and types of cancers do not appear unusual, the different types of cancers do not suggest a common exposure, and no exposures related to the types of cancers reported were identified.

The primary MF sources include the electrical panels, PDUs, and CUs. Secondary sources of MFs include the printers, tape drives, paper shredders, and portable heaters. The MFs are much greater when the electrical equipment is being operated or when electrical current is running through the equipment. Electrical current will always be running through the electrical panels and PDUs. In addition, the magnitude of the MFs will drop with increasing distance from the source.

All personal MF exposures were below applicable OELs with the exception of two peak exposures that were at or above the ACGIH ceiling limit of 1000 mG for employees with cardiac pacemakers or other electronic medical devices. Both of these peak exposures

DISCUSSION
(CONTINUED)

occurred in the computer server room. With the exception of the Computer Operator, all the GM personal exposures were below the GM exposures for similar job categories reported in the scientific literature [Bowman et al. 2008] and therefore may be considered typical for this type of work environment. The two employees who worked in the computer server room and adjacent areas had the highest GM exposure levels. For the other employees, peak exposures greater than 100 mG, with one exception, were traced back to activities in the computer server room.

These findings show that the MF exposure levels are related to movement patterns and the length of time spent in the computer server room, and for that reason are likely to vary from day to day. Because measurements were taken during a span of about 3 hours on one day, the range of typical exposures over time could not be determined. Nevertheless, the dominant source of the MFs on the day of the survey was the computer server room, and this is unlikely to change over time.

RECOMMENDATIONS

We recommend no further investigation into the cancers reported. The cancers among the Information Services Department employees are not likely to be due to their work. Nevertheless, employees may have concerns about their own risk for cancer. Therefore, management should take this opportunity to encourage employees to learn about the following:

- Known cancer risk factors

- Measures to reduce risk for preventable cancers

- Availability of cancer screening programs for certain types of cancer

The American Cancer Society posts information about cancer at www.cancer.org. For general information, click on "All about cancer" under "Patients, Family, & Friends." For information about a specific type of cancer, click on "Choose a cancer topic," select a type of cancer, then click "Go." Additionally, NIOSH posts information about occupational cancer and cancer cluster evaluations at www.cdc.gov/niosh/topics/cancer/.

Employees can take an active role in changing personal risk factors associated with certain types of cancer. In fact, the American

Cancer Society estimates that half of all cancer deaths in the United States were preventable [American Cancer Society 2008e]. In 2008, tobacco use alone caused an estimated 170,000 cancer deaths. It is well known that tobacco use is the single largest preventable cause of disease and increases the risk of 13 cancers including lung, mouth, nasal cavities, larynx, pharynx, esophagus, stomach, liver, pancreas, kidney, bladder, uterine cervix, and myeloid leukemia. High alcohol consumption, a diet low in fruits and vegetables, physical inactivity, overweight, and obesity are other modifiable personal risk factors that increase the risk of certain cancers. In fact, approximately one third of all cancer deaths in 2008 were related to poor nutrition, physical inactivity, and a high body mass index (a relationship between weight and height associated with body fat and health risk). Abundant scientific evidence shows that higher body mass indices are associated with an increased risk of 15 types of cancer including esophagus, stomach, colorectal, liver, gallbladder, pancreas, prostate, kidney, non-Hodgkin lymphoma, multiple myeloma, leukemia, breast, uterus, cervix, and ovary.

Another way for employees to prevent morbidity and mortality from cancer is to get cancer screening tests recommended for persons of their age and/or sex (e.g., colonoscopies for colon cancer screening, mammograms for breast cancer screening). Employees need to discuss available cancer screening programs with their primary care physicians. Screening can lead to earlier detection of cancers and earlier treatment, which may increase the chances of curing the disease.

The personal exposures measured in this survey did not exceed the ACGIH ceiling limit of 10000 mG. However, two of the peak exposures exceeded the ACGIH recommended ceiling limit of 1000 mG for employees with cardiac pacemakers or other similar electronic medical devices. The 10000 mG OEL is based on potential acute health effects; the 1000 mG OEL is based on potential interference with electronic medical devices. No OELs are based on the potential health effects from chronic MF exposures; however, exposures should be reduced whenever possible.

Because MFs cannot be easily shielded, administrative controls are the most feasible option to reduce the employees' exposures. Administrative controls are management-dictated work practices and policies to reduce or prevent exposures to workplace hazards. The effectiveness of administrative changes in work practices for controlling workplace hazards depends on management commitment and employee acceptance. Regular monitoring and reinforcement are necessary to ensure that control policies and procedures are not circumvented in the name of convenience or production. The following administrative controls are recommended to reduce the employees' personal exposures to the MFs.

1. Reduce the amount of time employees spend in the computer server room.

2. Encourage employees who must work in the computer server room to increase their working distance from the primary sources of the MFs. These sources include the electrical panel, PDUs, and CUs.

3. Do not allow employees with cardiac pacemakers or other similar electronic medical devices to enter the computer server room, as this room contains sources of MFs that could potentially exceed the ACGIH recommended ceiling limit of 1000 mG for such persons. A sign should be posted outside the computer server room that warns employees about the potential for MFs that interfere with the function of electronic medical devices. Employees using electronic medical devices should consult with their personal physician to determine if it is safe to enter the computer server room.

In addition, management and employees may want to learn more about MFs and other forms of EMF radiation. The following websites provide more information on occupational and environmental exposures, scientific research, and health concerns related to EMF radiation:

- NIOSH: www.cdc.gov/niosh/topics/emf/
- OSHA: www.osha.gov/SLTC/elfradiation/index.html
- WHO: www.who.int/peh-emf/en/
- NIEHS: www.niehs.nih.gov/health/topics/agents/emf/

REFERENCES

ACGIH [2008]. 2008 TLVs® and BEIs®: threshold limit values for chemical substances and physical agents and biological exposure indices. Cincinnati, OH: American Conference of Governmental Industrial Hygienists.

American Cancer Society [2006]. Occupation and cancer. [www.cancer.org/docroot/PRO/content/PRO_1_1x_Occupation_and_Cancer.pdf asp?sitearea=PRO]. Date accessed: January 9, 2009.

American Cancer Society [2008a]. Breast cancer facts and figures 2007–2008. [www.cancer.org/docroot/STT/stt_0_2007.asp?sitearea=STT&level=1]. Date accessed: January 9, 2009.

American Cancer Society [2008b]. Cancer facts and figures. [www.cancer.org/docroot/STT/content/STT_1x_Cancer_Facts_and_Figures_2008.asp?from=fast]. Date accessed: January 9, 2009.

American Cancer Society [2008c]. Prevention and early detection: secondhand smoke. [www.cancer.org/docroot/PED/content/PED_10_2X_Secondhand_Smoke-Clean_Indoor_Air.asp]. Date accessed: January 16, 2009.

American Cancer Society [2008d]. Detailed guide: pancreatic cancer. [www.cancer.org/docroot/CRI/CRI_2_1x.asp?rnav=criov&dt=34]. Date accessed: January 9, 2009.

American Cancer Society [2008e]. Cancer prevention and early detection facts & figures 2008. [http://www.cancer.org/docroot/STT/content/STT_1x_Cancer_Prevention_Early_Detection_Facts__Figures_2008.aspww]. Date accessed: January 9, 2009.

Bernstein L, Allen M, Anton-Culver H, Deapen D, Horn-Ross PL, Peel D, Pinder R, Reynolds P, Sullivan-Halley J, West D, Wright W, Ziogas A, Ross RK [2002]. High breast cancer incidence rates among California teachers: results from the California Teachers Study (United States). Cancer Causes Control 13(7):625–635.

Bowman J, Touchstone J, Yost M [2008]. Job exposure matrix for power-frequency magnetic fields. Cincinnati, OH: National Institute for Occupational Safety and Health [www.cdc.gov/niosh/topics/emf/jem-powerfreq/jempowerfreq.html]. Date accessed: January 8, 2009.

Calle EE, Murphy TK, Rodriguez C, Thun MJ, Heath CW [1998]. Occupation and breast cancer mortality in a prospective cohort of US women. Am J Epidemiol 148(2):191–197.

Carmichael A, Sami AS, Dixon JM [2003]. Breast cancer risk among the survivors of atomic bomb and patients exposed to therapeutic ionising radiation. Eur J Surg Oncol 29(5):475–479.

CDC (Centers for Disease Control) [1990]. Guidelines for investigating clusters of health events. MMWR 39(R-11):1–23.

Coogan PF, Clapp RW, Newcomb PA, Mittendorf R, Bogdan G, Baron JA, Longnecker MP [1996]. Variation in female breast cancer risk by occupation. Am J Ind Med 30(4):430–437.

EPA (Environmental Protection Agency) [2008]. Radon health risks. [www.epa.gov/radon/healthrisks.html]. Date accessed: January 16, 2009.

Feychting M, Forssen U [2006]. Electromagnetic fields and female breast cancer. Cancer Causes Control 17(4):553–558.

Goldberg MS, Labrèche F [1996]. Occupational risk factors for female breast cancer: a review. Occup Environ Med 53(3):145–156.

IARC [2002]. Monographs on the evaluation of the carcinogenic risks to humans: non-ionizing radiation, part 1: static and extremely low frequency electric and magnetic fields. Vol. 80. Lyon, France: World Health Organization, International Agency for Research on Cancer.

Kheifets L, Bowman JD, Checkoway H, Feychting M, Harrington M, Kavet R, Marsh G, Mezei G, Renew DC, van Wijngaarden E [2008]. Future needs of occupational epidemiology of extremely low frequency (ELF) electric and magnetic fields (EMF): review and recommendations. Occup Environ Med 66(2):72–80.

King AS, Threlfall WJ, Band PR, Gallagher RP [1994]. Mortality among female registered nurses and school teachers in British Columbia. Am J Ind Med 26(1):125–132.

MacArthur AC, Le ND, Abanto ZU, Gallagher RP [2007]. Occupational female breast and reproductive cancer mortality in British Columbia, Canada, 1950-94. Occup Med 57(4):246–253.

Metz LM, McGuinness S [1997]. Responding to reported clusters of common diseases: the case of multiple sclerosis. Can J Public Health 88(4):277–279.

Miller Y [2000]. Pulmonary neoplasms. In: Goldman L, Bennett J, eds. Cecil textbook of medicine. Philadelphia, PA: WB Saunders Co , pp. 449–455.

NIEHS [2002]. EMF electric and magnetic fields associated with the use of electric power. [www.niehs.nih.gov/health/topics/agents/emf/]. Date accessed: March 31, 2009.

Petralia SA, Vena JE, Freudenheim JL, Marshall JR, Michalek A, Brasure J, Swanson M, Graham S [1998]. Breast cancer risk and lifetime occupational history: employment in professional and managerial occupations. Occup Environ Med 55(1):43–48.

Pollán M, Gustavsson P [1999]. High-risk occupations for breast cancer in the Swedish female working population. Am J Public Health 89(6):875–881.

Rubin CH, Burnett CA, Halperin WE, Seligman PJ [1993]. Occupation as a risk identifier for breast cancer. Am J Public Health 83(9):1311–1315.

Rugo H [2004]. Occupational cancer. In: LaDou J, ed. Current occupational and environmental medicine. New York: McGraw Hill Companies, Inc , pp. 229–267.

Snedeker SM [2006]. Chemical exposures in the workplace: effect on breast cancer risk among women. AAOHN J 54(6):270–279.

Threlfall WJ, Gallagher RP, Spinelli JJ, Band PR [1985]. Reproductive variables as possible confounders in occupational studies of breast and ovarian cancer in females. J Occup Med 27(6):448–450.

Weiderpass E, Pukkala E, Kauppinen T, Mutanen P, Paakkulainen H, Vasama-Neuvonen K, Boffetta P, Partanen T [1999]. Breast cancer and occupational exposures in women in Finland. Am J Ind Med 36(1):48–53.

WHO [2002]. Establishing a dialog on risks from electromagnetic fields. Geneva, Switzerland: Radiation and Environmental Health,

REFERENCES
(CONTINUED)

Department of Protection of the Human Environment, World Health Organization.

WHO [2007]. Extremely low frequency fields. Environmental health criteria 238 Geneva: World Health Organization. [www.who.int/peh-emf/publications/elf_ehc/en/index.html]. Date accessed: January 10, 2009.

Zahl PH, Maehlen J, Welch HG [2008]. The natural history of invasive breast cancers detected by screening mammography. Arch Intern Med 168(21):2311–2316.

APPENDIX A: METHODS

MF measurements were collected using instruments that were calibrated within a month of the survey. Area measurements were collected using the HI-3627 ELF-MF Meter (Holaday Industries Inc., Eden Prairie, Minnesota). This meter is designed to measure the flux density of MFs in the frequency range of 5 to 2000 Hz. It computes the root mean square value of the 3-axis magnetic flux density and directly displays it on an analog meter. It is capable of measuring MF strength from 0.2 to 20000 mG, independently of the 3-axis probe orientation. Measurements were taken at a variety of locations throughout the workplace at a height of 48 inches to characterize levels near the torso of an employee.

Personal MF measurements were collected using the EMDEX II (Enertech Consultants, Campbell, California). This instrument is a programmable data-acquisition meter that measures the orthogonal-vector components of the MF through its internal sensors in the frequency range of 40 to 800 Hz. The instrument was set to record measurements every 1.5 seconds. Eight employees wore the meters on their waists for 3 or more hours during the morning. Four employees volunteered to wear the meters, including the two employees who worked in the computer server room. The other employees were selected by us according to their job title and office location to obtain a representative sample of the employee population.

APPENDIX B: OCCUPATIONAL EXPOSURE LIMITS AND HEALTH EFFECTS

In evaluating the hazards posed by workplace exposures, NIOSH investigators use both mandatory (legally enforceable) and recommended OELs for chemical, physical, and biological agents as a guide for making recommendations. OELs have been developed by Federal agencies and safety and health organizations to prevent the occurrence of adverse health effects from workplace exposures. Generally, OELs suggest levels of exposure to which most employees may be exposed up to 10 hours per day, 40 hours per week for a working lifetime without experiencing adverse health effects. However, not all employees will be protected from adverse health effects even if their exposures are maintained below these levels. A small percentage may experience adverse health effects because of individual susceptibility, a pre-existing medical condition, and/or a hypersensitivity (allergy). In addition, some hazardous substances may act in combination with other workplace exposures, the general environment, or with medications or personal habits of the employee to produce health effects even if the occupational exposures are controlled at the level set by the exposure limit. Also, some substances can be absorbed by direct contact with the skin and mucous membranes in addition to being inhaled, which contributes to the individual's overall exposure.

Most OELs are expressed as a TWA exposure. A TWA refers to the average exposure during a normal 8- to 10-hour workday. Some chemical substances and physical agents have recommended STEL or ceiling values where health effects are caused by exposures over a short period. Unless otherwise noted, the STEL is a 15-minute TWA exposure that should not be exceeded at any time during a workday, and the ceiling limit is an exposure that should not be exceeded at any time.

In the United States, OELs have been established by Federal agencies, professional organizations, state and local governments, and other entities. Some OELs are legally enforceable limits, while others are recommendations. The U.S. Department of Labor OSHA PELs (29 CFR 1910 [general industry]; 29 CFR 1926 [construction industry]; and 29 CFR 1917 [maritime industry]) are legal limits enforceable in workplaces covered under the Occupational Safety and Health Act. NIOSH RELs are recommendations based on a critical review of the scientific and technical information available on a given hazard and the adequacy of methods to identify and control the hazard. NIOSH RELs can be found in the *NIOSH Pocket Guide to Chemical Hazards* [NIOSH 2005]. NIOSH also recommends different types of risk management practices (e.g., engineering controls, safe work practices, employee education/training, personal protective equipment, and exposure and medical monitoring) to minimize the risk of exposure and adverse health effects from these hazards. Other OELs that are commonly used and cited in the United States include the TLVs recommended by ACGIH, a professional organization, and the WEELs recommended by the American Industrial Hygiene Association, another professional organization. The TLVs and WEELs are developed by committee members of these associations from a review of the published, peer-reviewed literature. They are not consensus standards. ACGIH TLVs are considered voluntary exposure guidelines for use by industrial hygienists and others trained in this discipline "to assist in the control of health hazards" [ACGIH 2008]. WEELs have been established for some chemicals "when no other legal or authoritative limits exist" [AIHA 2008].

Outside the United States, OELs have been established by various agencies and organizations and include both legal and recommended limits. Since 2006, the Berufsgenossenschaftliches Institut für Arbeitsschutz (German Institute for Occupational Safety and Health) has maintained a database of international OELs from European Union member states, Canada (Québec), Japan, Switzerland, and the United States available at www.hvbg.de/e/bia/gestis/limit_values/index.html. The database contains international limits for over 1250 hazardous substances and is updated annually.

Employers should understand that not all hazardous chemicals have specific OSHA PELs, and for some agents the legally enforceable and recommended limits may not reflect current health-based information. However, an employer is still required by OSHA to protect its employees from hazards even in the absence of a specific OSHA PEL. OSHA requires an employer to furnish employees a place of employment free from recognized hazards that cause or are likely to cause death or serious physical harm [Occupational Safety and Health Act of 1970 (Public Law 91–596, sec. 5(a)(1))]. Thus, NIOSH investigators encourage employers to make use of other OELs when making risk assessment and risk management decisions to best protect the health of their employees. NIOSH investigators also encourage the use of the traditional hierarchy of controls approach to eliminate or minimize identified workplace hazards. This includes, in order of preference, the use of (1) substitution or elimination of the hazardous agent, (2) engineering controls (e.g , local exhaust ventilation, process enclosure, dilution ventilation), (3) administrative controls (e.g., limiting time of exposure, employee training, work practice changes, medical surveillance), and (4) personal protective equipment (e.g., respiratory protection, gloves, eye protection, hearing protection). Control banding, a qualitative risk assessment and risk management tool, is a complementary approach to protecting employee health that focuses resources on exposure controls by describing how a risk needs to be managed. Information on control banding is available at www.cdc.gov/niosh/topics/ctrlbanding/. This approach can be applied in situations where OELs have not been established or can be used to supplement the OELs, when available.

Magnetic Fields

Although OSHA and NIOSH have not established OELs for MFs in the extremely low frequency range (3 to 3000 Hz), several organizations have, including the American National Standards Institute, the Institute of Electrical and Electronics Engineers, and the ACGIH. Among these organizations, the ACGIH has published frequency-dependent TLVs. Because the MFs at the Information Services Department come primarily from 60 Hz power lines, the whole-body TLV ceiling limit of 10000 mG applies. The health and safety basis for this TLV is that MFs greater than this level can induce currents in the body and cause magnetophosphenes in the visual system [ACGIH 2006]. The ACGIH also recommends a power frequency ceiling limit of 1000 mG for employees wearing cardiac pacemakers or similar medical electronic devices to protect against the interference with the function of these devices [ACGIH 2008]. Neither the TLV, nor any of the other OELs, address potential health effects from chronic MF exposures.

Much research has been conducted during the past decade to determine if slightly elevated MF exposures (greater than 2 mG) pose a health threat. The NIEHS evaluated many of these studies and, in 1999, concluded that "... the probability that EMF exposure is truly a health hazard is currently small. The weak epidemiological associations provide only marginal, scientific support that exposure to this agent is causing any degree of harm." However, the report also states that EMF exposures "cannot be recognized as entirely safe" and that efforts should continue to reduce exposures [NIEHS 1999]. More recently, in 2002, the IARC classified extremely low frequency MFs as possibly carcinogenic to humans based on epidemiology studies of childhood leukemia. This classification is used to denote an agent that has limited evidence of carcinogenicity in humans and less than sufficient evidence for carcinogenicity in experimental animals. Evidence for all other cancers in children and adults was inadequate to classify due to insufficient or inconsistent scientific information [IARC 2002]. A 2007 update of this evaluation did not change the classification based upon more recent studies [WHO 2007].

References

ACGIH [2006]. Sub-radiofrequency (30 KHz and below) magnetic fields. In: Documentation of the threshold limit values and biological exposure indices. Cincinnati, OH: American Conference of Governmental Industrial Hygienists.

ACGIH [2008]. 2008 TLVs® and BEIs®: threshold limit values for chemical substances and physical agents and biological exposure indices. Cincinnati, OH: American Conference of Governmental Industrial Hygienists.

AIHA [2008]. AIHA 2008 Emergency response planning guidelines (ERPG) & workplace environmental exposure levels (WEEL) handbook. Fairfax, VA: American Industrial Hygiene Association.

CFR. Code of Federal Regulations. Washington, DC: U.S. Government Printing Office, Office of the Federal Register.

IARC [2002]. Monographs on the evaluation of the carcinogenic risks to humans: non-ionizing radiation, part 1: static and extremely low frequency electric and magnetic fields. Vol. 80. Lyon, France: World Health Organization, International Agency for Research on Cancer.

NIEHS [1999]. NIEHS report on health effects from exposure to power-line frequency electric and magnetic fields. By Boorman G, Bernheim N, Galvin M, Newton S, Parham F, Portier C, Wolfe M. Research Triangle Park, NC: U.S. Department of Health and Human Services, National Institutes of Health, National Institute for Environmental Health Sciences (NIEHS) Publication No. 99-4493.

NIOSH [2005]. NIOSH pocket guide to chemical hazards. Cincinnati, OH: U.S. Department of Health and Human Services, Centers for Disease Control and Prevention, National Institute for Occupational Safety and Health, DHHS (NIOSH) Publication No. 2005-149. [www.cdc.gov/niosh/npg/]. Date accessed: March 2008.

WHO [2007]. Extremely low frequency fields. Environmental health criteria 238 Geneva: World Health Organization [www.who.int/peh-emf/publications/elf_ehc/en/index.html]. Date accessed: January 10, 2009.

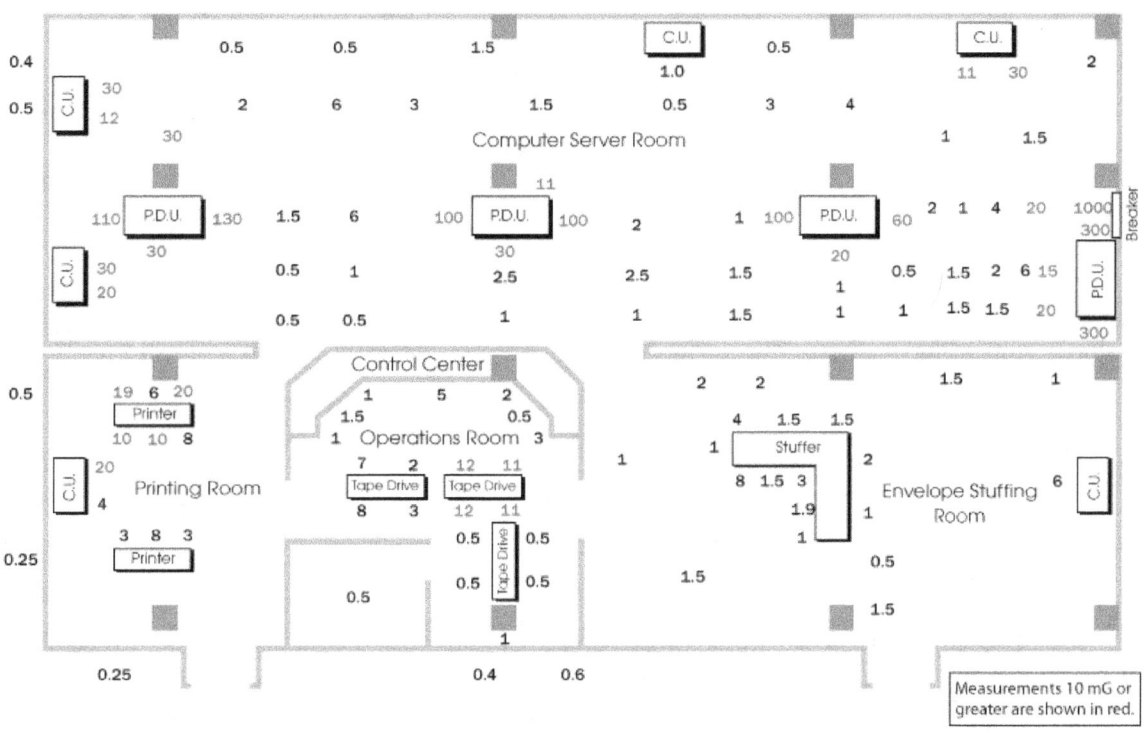

Figure 2. MF levels (mG) measured in the computer server room, printing room, operations room, and envelope stuffing room

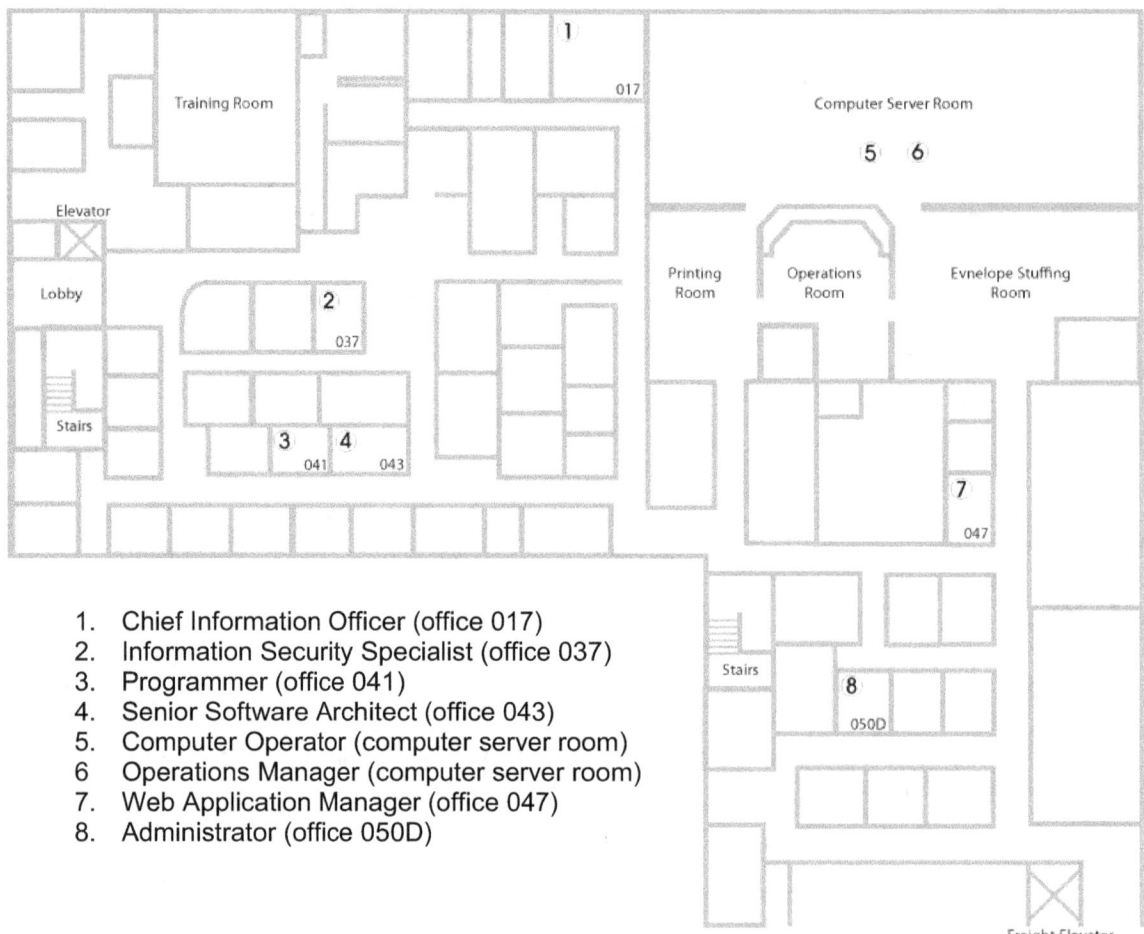

1. Chief Information Officer (office 017)
2. Information Security Specialist (office 037)
3. Programmer (office 041)
4. Senior Software Architect (office 043)
5. Computer Operator (computer server room)
6. Operations Manager (computer server room)
7. Web Application Manager (office 047)
8. Administrator (office 050D)

Figure 3. Work station locations for employees who wore personal monitors

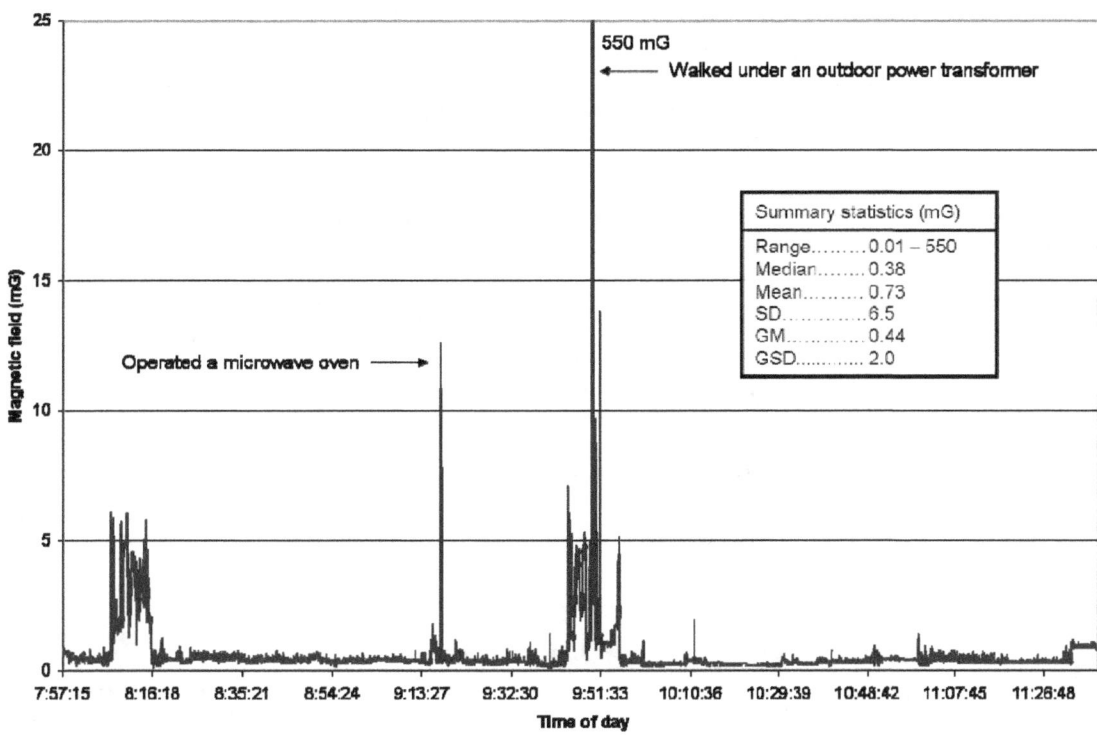

Figure 4. Personal MF exposures over time for the Programmer

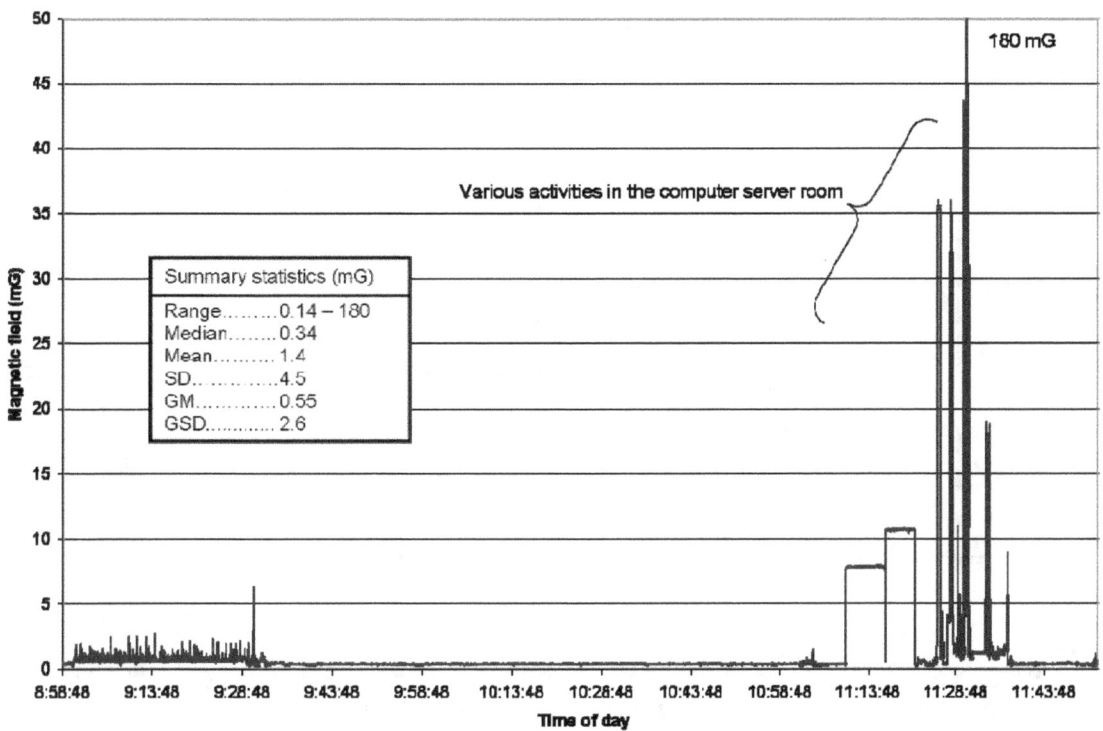

Figure 5. Personal MF exposures over time for the Administrator

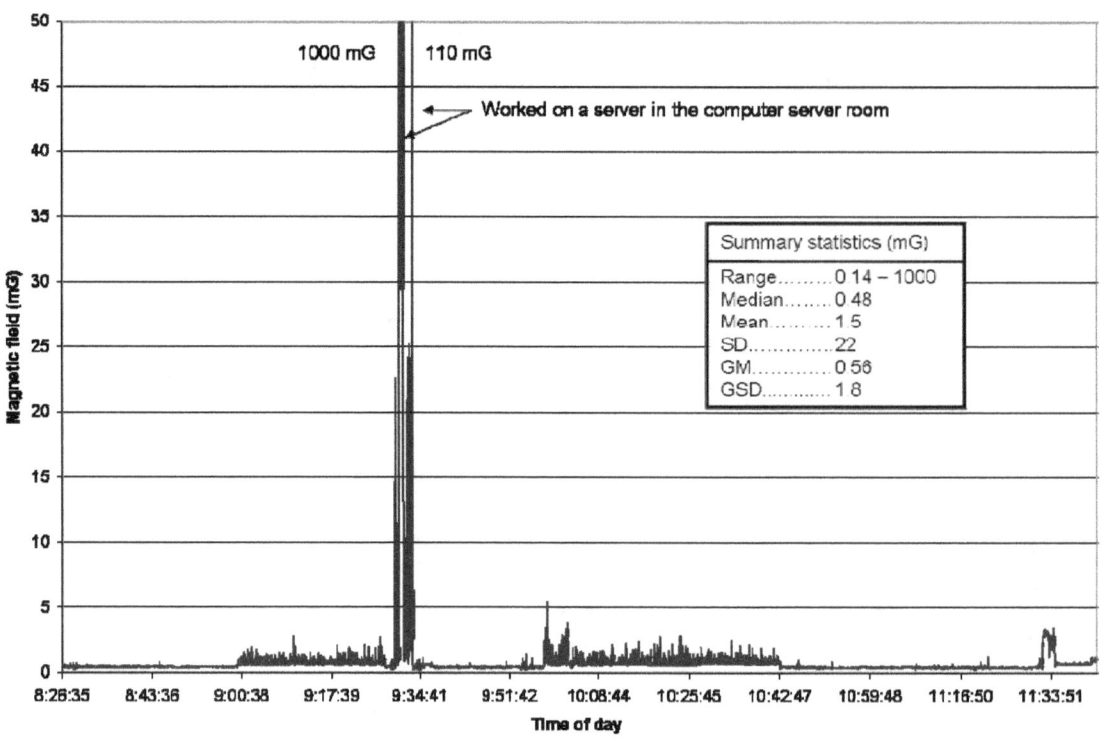

Figure 6. Personal MF exposures over time for the Chief Information Officer

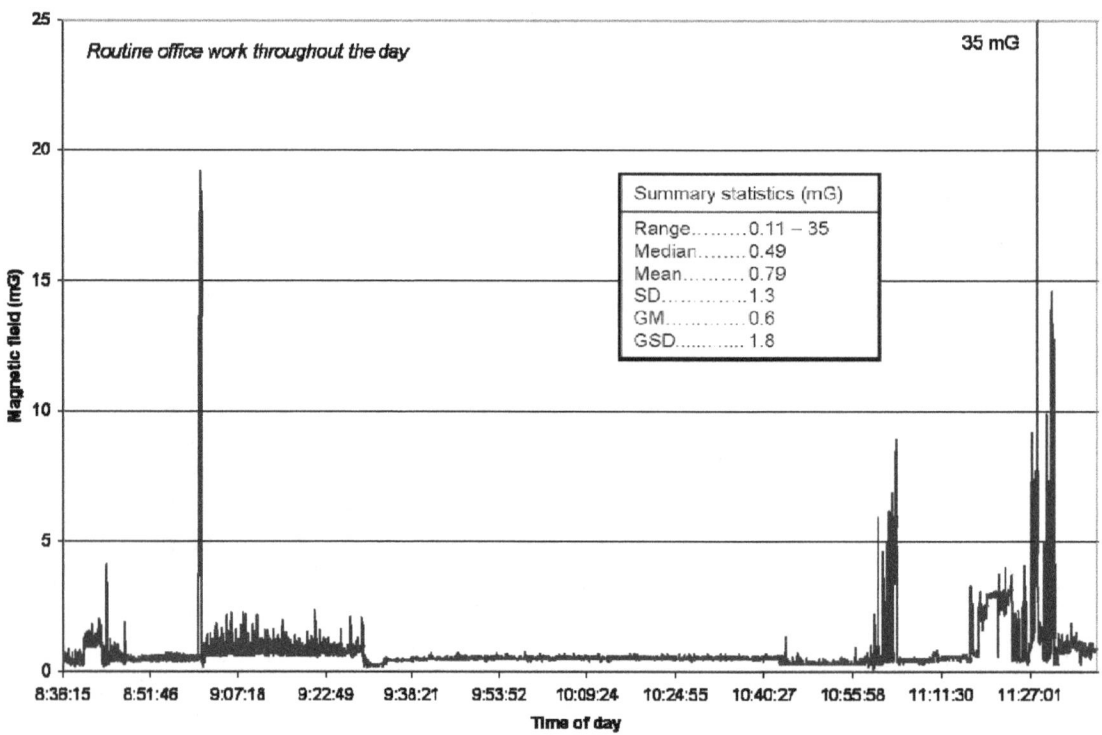

Figure 7. Personal MF exposures over time for the Information Security Specialist

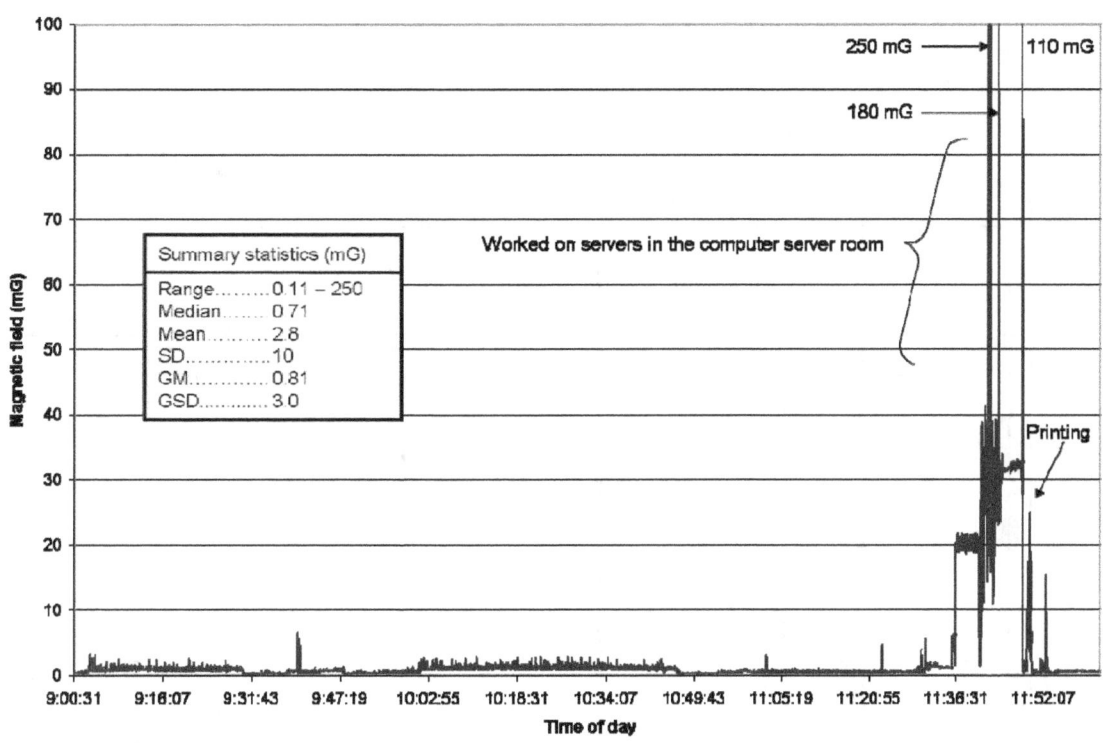

Figure 8. Personal MF exposures over time for the Senior Software Architect

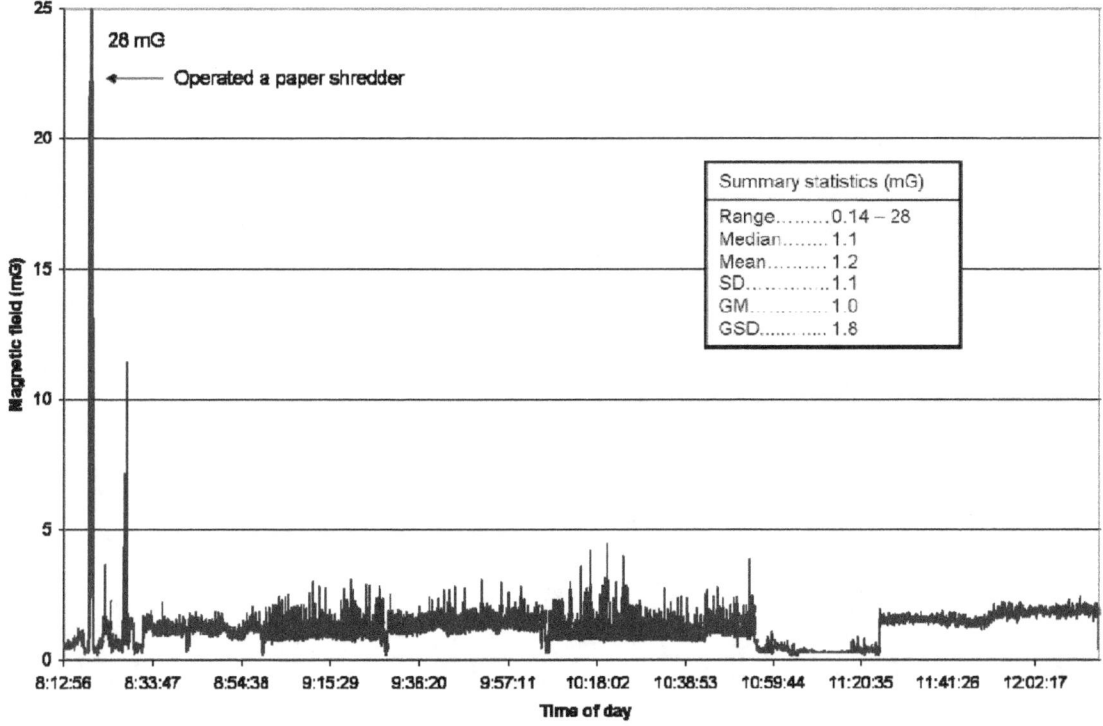

Figure 9. Personal MF exposures over time for the Web Application Manager

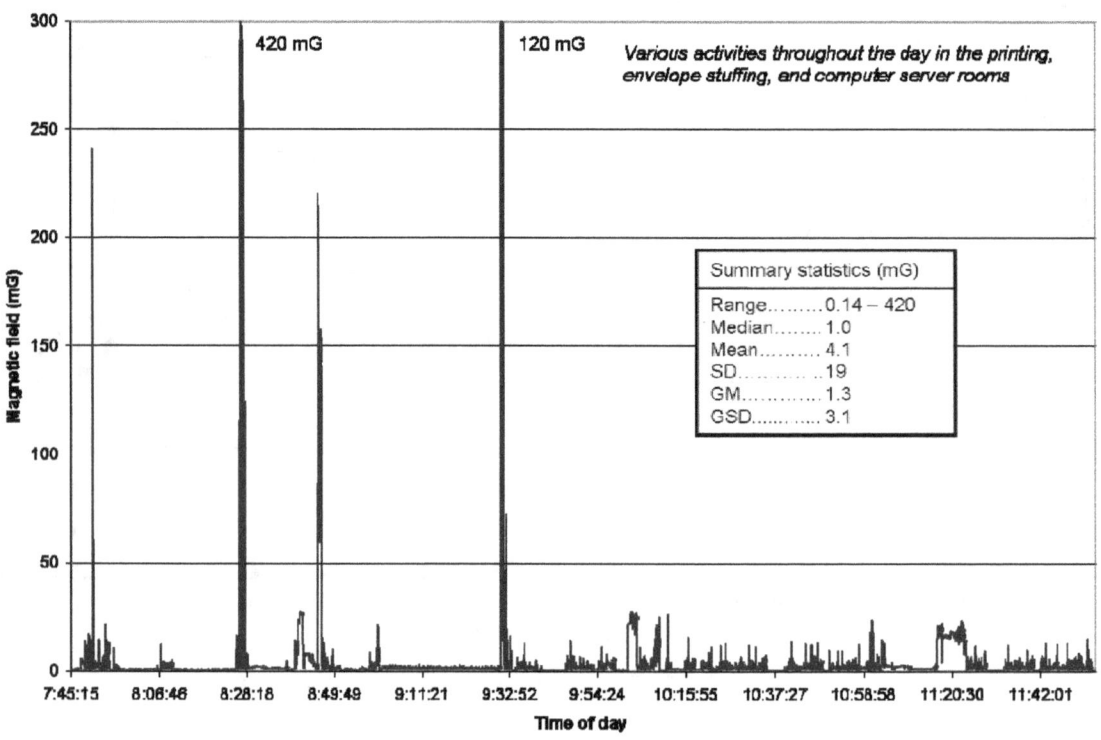

Figure 10. Personal MF exposures over time for the Operations Manager

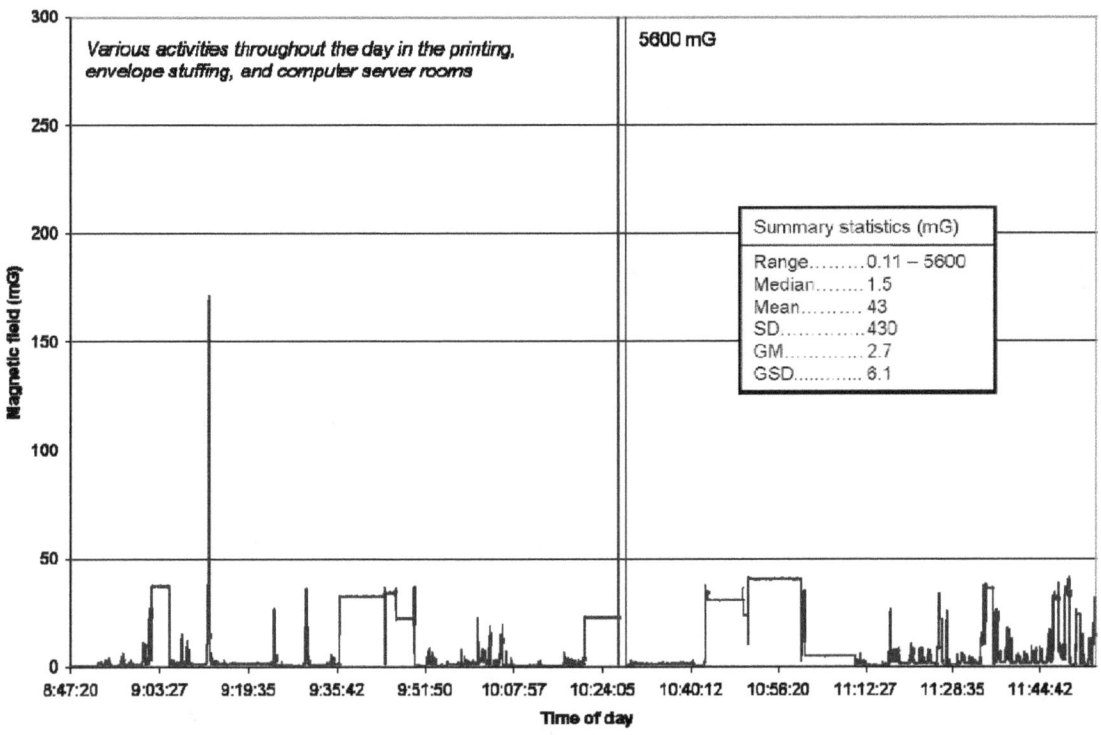

Figure 11. Personal MF exposures over time for the Computer Operator

This page intentionally left blank

Acknowledgments and Availability of Report

The Hazard Evaluations and Technical Assistance Branch (HETAB) of the National Institute for Occupational Safety and Health (NIOSH) conducts field investigations of possible health hazards in the workplace. These investigations are conducted under the authority of Section 20(a)(6) of the Occupational Safety and Health (OSHA) Act of 1970, 29 U.S.C. 669(a)(6) which authorizes the Secretary of Health and Human Services, following a written request from any employer or authorized representative of employees, to determine whether any substance normally found in the place of employment has potentially toxic effects in such concentrations as used or found. HETAB also provides, upon request, technical and consultative assistance to federal, state, and local agencies; labor; industry; and other groups or individuals to control occupational health hazards and to prevent related trauma and disease.

The findings and conclusions in this report are those of the authors and do not necessarily represent the views of NIOSH. Mention of any company or product does not constitute endorsement by NIOSH. In addition, citations to websites external to NIOSH do not constitute NIOSH endorsement of the sponsoring organizations or their programs or products. Furthermore, NIOSH is not responsible for the content of these websites. All Web addresses referenced in this document were accessible as of the publication date.

This report was prepared by Kenneth W. Fent and Elena Page of HETAB, Division of Surveillance, Hazard Evaluations and Field Studies. Industrial hygiene field assistance was provided by Greg Burr. Medical field assistance was provided by Nancy Williams. Health communication assistance was provided by Stefanie Evans. Editorial assistance was provided by Ellen Galloway. Desktop publishing was performed by Robin Smith.

Copies of this report have been sent to employee and management representatives at the County of Guilford, Information Services Department; and the OSHA Regional Office. This report is not copyrighted and may be freely reproduced. The report may be viewed and printed at www.cdc.gov/niosh/hhe. Copies may be purchased from the National Technical Information Service at 5825 Port Royal Road, Springfield, Virginia 22161.

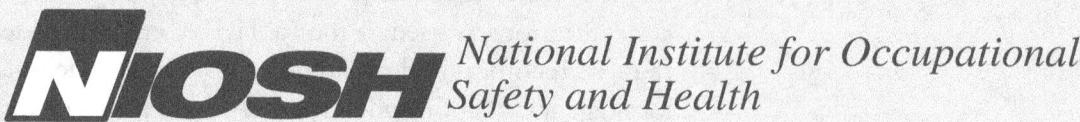 *National Institute for Occupational Safety and Health*

Delivering on the Nation's promise: Safety and health at work for all people through research and prevention.

To receive NIOSH documents or information about occupational safety and health topics, contact NIOSH at:

1-800-CDC-INFO (1-800-232-4636)

TTY: 1-888-232-6348

E-mail: cdcinfo@cdc.gov

or visit the NIOSH web site at: **www.cdc.gov/niosh.**

For a monthly update on news at NIOSH, subscribe to NIOSH eNews by visiting **www.cdc.gov/niosh/eNews.**

SAFER • HEALTHIER • PEOPLE™